MINDFULNESS MEDITATION: A BEGINNER'S GUIDE TO YOGA MEDITATION

How to Relieve Stress and Find Happiness in Your Life

by George M. Posi

Table of contents

INTRODUCTION

I want to thank you and congratulate you on reading the book "Mindfulness Meditation: A Beginner's Guide to Yoga Meditation." This book contains proven steps and strategies for how to relieve stress, find happiness in your life, create your inner peace, and make your life better.

Mindfulness meditation will help you to remain calm and in the present moment. You will learn to live in this moment. You do not have control over your past or your future. Mindfulness meditation teaches you the importance of what you are doing now and space through which you are moving at each moment.

Bottom line: mindfulness is the practice of focusing all your attention on the present moment purposefully and accepting it resolutely without judgment. It's a perfect place to begin if you are looking for true peace and happiness.

Meditative techniques are an essential part of any yoga exercise. Even though you don't need to formally meditate to practice yoga, the two practices support each other. Through your practice of yoga, you enhance both your ability to concentrate and to relax. Those are the two most essential requirements for meditation practice. Here, you can deepen your understanding of what meditation is and begin a practice of your own.

Thanks again for reading this book. I hope you enjoy it!

WHAT IS MEDITATION?

It is known from ancient times that mindfulness meditation is a powerful technique. It has been used for thousands of years to reduce anxiety, depression, stress, and help you achieve peace of mind.

Mindfulness meditation helps you train your mind to remain in the present moment, entirely calm and aware of your surroundings. Often, we become anxious and stressed because of a troubling past that we still think about or being upset about a future that is yet to come and that we have no control over. With mindfulness meditation, you will learn to live in only the present moment.

The practices of mindfulness meditation originate from Hinduism. Buddhism has adopted these techniques and improved on them, so they become integral to what is referred to as the "Buddhist path." In Buddhism, cultivating non-judgmental awareness of yourself, your feelings, and your mind is considered crucial if you want to lead a calm and peaceful life.

What is most important for the mind is to fully attend to what is taking place, to what you are doing, and to space through which you are moving. If we stop being in touch with our body and become absorbed in obsessive thoughts about stuff that has already taken place or if we always worry about the future, then we create anxiety for ourselves. Even in such moments, mindfulness is there to take us back to where we are and what we are feeling and doing.

In the yoga tradition, there is a methodology that is designed to show us the connection between every living thing. Meditation is the actual experience of this union (Advaita).

Instructions for how to meditate and description of meditation practice are found in the Yoga Sutra. This mental stillness brings the body, mind, and senses into a state of balance. This also relaxes the nervous system. Real meditation begins after we realize that our need to possess and our everlasting craving for pleasure will never be satisfied. Only then does our external pursuit turn inward, and we are in the real state of meditation. Meditation (Dhyana) in the yogic context is defined as a state of pure consciousness. When we are aware of our senses but disengaged at the same time. Our concentration allowed us to be grounded, mentally, and physically. In fact, meditation is much more than concentration. It represents an expanded state of awareness.

To achieve the state of self-realization (Samadhi), it is not enough just to focus our mind on an object apart from ourselves. We need to do more than only establish contact and get familiar with it. We need to communicate with this object and gain a deep awareness of the fact that there is no difference between this object and ourselves.

When we are separate from nature, we feel pain and suffering, according to the Yoga Sutra. To stay in contact with nature, we can make our minds stable and focused, and we can make full use of it and enable our consciousness to grow. This is best accomplished through the practice of mindfulness meditation. When you meditate, you use a technique to develop your mind, the same way you use physical exercise to build your muscles.

We all have a restless mind. Thoughts just come uninvited at any moment of the day and even at night. This is a waste of your precious mental energy, and as such, you get exhausted by these wandering thoughts. Meditation will help you to eliminate those thoughts.

How does meditation work?

The word "meditation" does not describe all Buddhist ideas embodied in the Pali word "Bhavana." It means much more and can be defined as "to develop our mental ability." Meditation is more than be willing to sit quietly and close your eyes. It is more than thinking about only the good things in your life and disregarding all that is bad. It is not about becoming overly optimistic. Meditation has everything to do with your everyday life. It is not only for monks and old people who have retired and have time for it.

In the Buddhist teachings, we learn to recognize six senses. The outside world is brought to us through the eyes, ears, nose, tongue, body, and mind. The first five are physical senses, and the mind works as a mental sense. Things you perceive through your six senses are meditation objects.

This knowledge of how to perceive the world is essential for successful meditation.

THE BENEFITS OF MEDITATION

Herbert Benson, MD, a researcher at Harvard University Medical School, found that relaxation is not the goal of meditation, but that it is often a result. The relaxation response, as he called it, is "an opposite, involuntary response that causes a reduction in the activity of the sympathetic nervous system."

Various studies on the relaxation response have also found the benefits of reducing activity in the nervous system:

- Lower blood pressure
- Improved blood circulation
- Lower heart rate
- Less perspiration
- Slower respiratory rate
- Less anxiety
- Lower blood cortisol levels
- More feelings of satisfied well-being
- Less stress
- Deeper relaxation

Those are mainly short-term benefits, but some researchers suspect that there are some long-term benefits as well. But remember that the purpose of meditation is not to achieve any benefits from it. Be present in this moment and at this place is the ultimate goal of meditation.

According to Buddhist teachings, the mind being free from attachment is the ultimate benefit of meditation. Letting go of things our mind cannot control and maintaining the sense of inner harmony are the keys to the path of achieving true liberation. Our mind will learn how to stop needlessly following desires or clinging to experiences and thus become genuinely calm.

Research has confirmed that profound psychological and physiological changes happen when we meditate. Meditation changes specific processes in the brain and other involuntary processes of the body.

Meditation helps you to manage stress. Reducing stress improves your overall physical health and emotional well-being. Meditation raises the quality of your life by teaching you to be fully alert, aware, and alive. In fact, we are not meditating to gain something. We meditate to let go of things that we don't need.

TYPES OF MEDITATION

There are many different types of meditation. You should try some of them and decide which is your favorite, which one works the best for you. Do your research and tests, but do not give up easily. For you to know if this is the right technique for you, you must let it settle, let it become a part of your routine. If you are not satisfied with the feelings provided by this type of meditative practice after a few weeks, try something different.

Here are some of the main types of meditative practices, but remember that there are a lot of variations on all of them.

Mindfulness with Breathing Meditation

In this type of meditation, you will start with a breath. You will learn how different types of breathing have different effects on your body. We will explain the posture and place for meditation. Let me just tell you that the site for your meditation practice does not need to be perfect because you cannot find such an area. No place is perfect.

It is important to sit in a way that is both stable and secure, so when the mind becomes semiconscious, you will not fall over. It is also important to sit upright, with the vertebrae and spine in proper alignment, without any bends or curves. The vertebrae should sit snugly, one on top of the other, so that they fit together correctly.

At first, keep your eyes open, gazing toward the tip of your nose so that your eyes do not get involved with other distractions. If you close your eyes, you might get sleepy, so be careful about this option. Later, as you gain more experience, you will be able to meditate even with your eyes closed—without falling asleep.

Let your breath be natural. Do not interfere with it in any way. Then, contemplate each breath with mindfulness. How are you breathing? What is exhale like? Note your observations so you can compare them with your later experiences.

It also helps to count. You can count each inhalation as it starts, one number for each breath. If your mind wanders, start counting again. If you can count to ten without the mind wandering, go back to the count of "one" anyway.

These tricks will help you get started. When you adopt them, you will always have them at your service in your meditation and in your everyday life.

Metta Meditation

As a part of your meditation routine, you can focus your inner attention on someone you know who might benefit from an extra dose of kindness and care. Send this person love, happiness, and well-being. In the Buddhist tradition, this is called Metta meditation practice, and it can benefit you greatly.

"Metta" can be translated from Pali (the language of Buddha) as "loving-kindness" or "friendly love." Many Buddhists regard this type of meditation as the default kind. Metta meditation is constructed of four components: Metta, Karuna (compassion), Mudita (sympathetic joy), and Upekkha (balanced mind).

Metta represents the desire to see peace and success in your life, as well as to be free from harm. This then extends to members of your family and friends, and later, it becomes universal.

For Metta meditation to be successful, you must have engaged in putting forth the right effort. You must really mean the words that you are saying to yourself while meditating. Developing Metta —developing loving-kindness toward yourself— is, therefore, crucial in overcoming frustration within oneself. This gradual reduction of frustration is the first benefit that one earns from Metta meditation.

In the beginning, choose yourself as the meditation object. Repeat to yourself in your thoughts, "May I be free from (state first negative condition). May I be free from (other negative condition). May I be able to (state first positive condition). May I be able to (other negative condition)." Repeat these two to five times.

You will next dedicate your thoughts to people you care about: your parents, children, spouse, or siblings. Visualize them and repeat: "May they be free from (say your choice of one negative condition). May they be free from (say your choice of a second negative condition). May they be able to (say your choice of a positive condition). May they be able to (say your choice of a second positive condition)." You can wish them to be free from illness, and to have good health, or some more specific condition that you know is appropriate for them.

In this way, you will develop mindfulness of your feelings of well-being, your desire to be free from harm, and suffering, and this then leads to the development of Metta for yourself and the people closest to you.

Now, you choose a neutral person. They may be someone from work or someone you have come across anywhere you've gone, someone you neither like nor dislike. This person is entirely neutral. Direct your Metta thoughts to that person in the same way as you did before.

In your first Metta meditations, do not use the people you have been in conflict with or had arguments with. Do not start with people of the gender you're attracted to, as this can provoke lust. Also, do not use those who have died, for this can stir up sorrow.

You can also have the next part of Metta meditation directed to an unspecified person (your whole country, world, any other living being, etc.). You can try doing this in your next meditations.

Vipassana Meditation

The purpose of meditation is to clear your mind and get rid of greed, hatred, and jealousy. Meditation helps you to bring your mind to a state of concentration, insight, and tranquility, and by doing so, you can achieve awareness.

You might like to practice Vipassana meditation to help you face reality or to experience life just as it is. After that, you can change the way you live

You must learn to listen to your own thoughts without getting caught up in them. That way, you will see the truth: objects are impermanent and unsatisfactory.

By practicing Vipassana meditation, you will be able to condition yourself to see reality truly as it is. You will gain mindfulness.

There is no unique technique to it. You are practicing Vipassana when you focus on breathing—just letting any emotions, feelings, and thoughts to arise. You acknowledge them, accept them, and then let them go. You just need to sit and genuinely commit to doing Vipassana meditation.

Other Forms of Meditation

Within the Judeo-Christian tradition, there are two leading practices: prayer and contemplation. Prayer can be described as an address to God.

Contemplation is a process of conscious thought about a specific topic, like a religious ideal or religious script. Prayer and reflection are exercises in concentration.

Hindu tradition treats yogic meditation as purely concentrative. It focuses the mind on a single object, not allowing it to wander. In advanced practice, yogis proceed to expand it by assuming more complex objects of meditation.

In addition to concentration, Buddhist meditation aims toward the development of awareness, using concentration only as a tool toward that end. The aim of Zen Buddhist meditation is to just sit down and throw everything out of your mind. You keep only the pure awareness of sitting. This is very hard to achieve.

On the other side of "toughness" is Tantric Buddhism. So, there are many ways to achieve peace of mind.

MEDITATION IN MOTION

While I was at a Suan Mokkh meditation retreat in Chaiya, Thailand, I had the opportunity to try different types of meditative practice (like yoga, Taiji, or Qigong). This group that I particularly like can be called "meditation in motion." Every morning, we had one of these practices, and I must say that I feel that by beginning the day in mindful motion, your whole day starts developing in a much more positive fashion.

Taiji (Tai Chi)

Taiji (tai chi), is a Chinese martial art practiced not only for its physical but also for its health benefits and meditation practices. It is another excellent example of the meditation-in-motion concept. In its movement, Taiji practice embodies the philosophy of yin and yang.

In the latest period, Taiji has developed worldwide recognition, with the focus on improving personal physical and mental health.

Focusing your mind on the movements helps you achieve calm and clarity of the mind. Again, according to Wikipedia, it is "considered to teach the use of leverage through the joints based on coordination and relaxation, rather than muscular tension, to neutralize, yield, or initiate attacks. The slow, repetitive work involved in the process of learning how that leverage is generated gently and [how it] measurably increases, as well as opens, the internal circulation (breath, body heat, blood, lymph, peristalsis)."

One may say that Taiji is both health training and meditation practice, along with its original martial art component.

Qigong

"Qigong" is pronounced "Chi-Gung."

"Qigong is a holistic system of coordinated body posture and movement, breathing, and meditation used for the purposes of health, spirituality, and martial arts training. With roots in Chinese medicine, philosophy, and martial arts, Qigong is traditionally viewed by the Chinese and throughout Asia as a practice to cultivate and balance qi (pronounced approximately as "chi"), translated as "life energy" (Wikipedia).

Deep rhythmic breathing, slow-flowing movement, and a calm meditative state of mind are the focuses of Qigong practice and philosophy.

The core of Qigong contains practices that coordinate body, breath, and mind. It has its origins in Chinese philosophy. Qigong practice consists of both moving and still meditation in various postures, massage, and chanting, etc. As it is primarily a form of moving meditation, Qigong practice involves carefully choreographed movement, coordinated with breath and awareness.

Yoga

For thousands of years, yoga has been one of the most effective ways to manage stress, gain happiness, and establish peace of mind. It can also help to reduce body pain, as well as increase flexibility and body strength.

In Sanskrit, the word "yoga" is usually used to signify connection or union. Yoga is actually the whole process of being more aware of who you are.

The origin of yoga can be traced back to more than 5,000 years ago in northern India. In the oldest sacred texts known as the Rig Veda, we find the first reference to the word "yoga." This text contained mantras, rituals, and songs used by the Vedic priests (Brahmans).

In a broad sense, yoga represents a group of physical, mental, and spiritual practices. In the Western world, it is often simplified to assume physical exercise postures (asanas), mainly referring to Hatha yoga. Even though texts about Hatha yoga date from between the 9th and 11th centuries, with origins in tantra, it is only in the 19th and 20th centuries that yoga became known to Westerners.

As stated on Wikipedia, "Yoga as exercise is a physical activity consisting largely of asanas, often connected by flowing sequences called Vinyasas, sometimes accompanied by the breathing exercises of Pranayama, and usually ending with a period of relaxation or meditation."

It is often forgotten that the goals of yoga are spiritual liberation, achieving inner peace, and being in harmony with nature. Meditation is a spiritual part of yoga that cannot be set apart. That why we sometimes refer to yoga practice as "meditation in motion."

The Connection Between Yoga and Meditation

In today's hectic world, we look for activities that help us calm our minds. We know from our experience that techniques to calm your mind can help fight anxiety and improve our mood. We call those activities "mindfulness."

It is accepted that not only does yoga help to fight depression, but it also improves your physical well-being. Regular practice lightens your mood and takes you away from your everyday troubles, even if just for that moment when we practice. A combination of physical and mental incentives that yoga offers should be embraced and broadened by regular practice. It will help you to manage stress effectively.

Yoga also helps your sense of accomplishment after you finish your daily yoga routine. It also prepares you to enter deeper states of mind by practicing breathing (Pranayama) and performing different meditative methods inside your yoga practice. Yoga postures are intended to prepare your body for meditation.

When we begin to slow our breath and begin to sync it with our movement, we become calm. Then, we grow closer to the single-minded purpose. By slowing down, we begin to accomplish more, and we keep our attention in the present moment. Yoga not only helps to strengthen our body, but raises our awareness, and prepares us for meditation. Proper breathing helps calm your mind. It gives a rhythm to your thoughts and helps create a peaceful structure of the mind.

Meditation and yoga are interrelated. Yogis say, "Where the breath flows, the mind goes." Yoga, like meditative chanting, can allow the energy to flow upward and to open our heart to the higher chakras and higher consciousness.

Shavasana, the Yoga Meditation for Relaxation

The most popular pose in yoga for meditation practice is Shavasana (corpse pose). It is practically the most integral part of any yoga class. Though yoga is often described as "Moving Meditation," this pose requires you to be completely calm and still, thus entering a meditative state.

The word "Shavasana" has Sanskrit origins. We practice the Shavasana pose by lying face-up on the ground, arms and legs comfortably spread, and with eyes closed. To begin, we will gradually scan our body down from head to toe, relaxing one body part at a time. Keep awareness of the parts of the body that feel relaxed. Notice which parts are still tense.

Do you feel comfortable or uncomfortable? Is your body light or heavy? If thoughts arise, just notice them and let your breath carry them away. Let your breath bring you to the place of stillness. The more you practice, the easier it gets to achieve this. In time, your breathing will become quieter, slower, and more profound. You will become really calm, not only when practicing but in your everyday life as well.

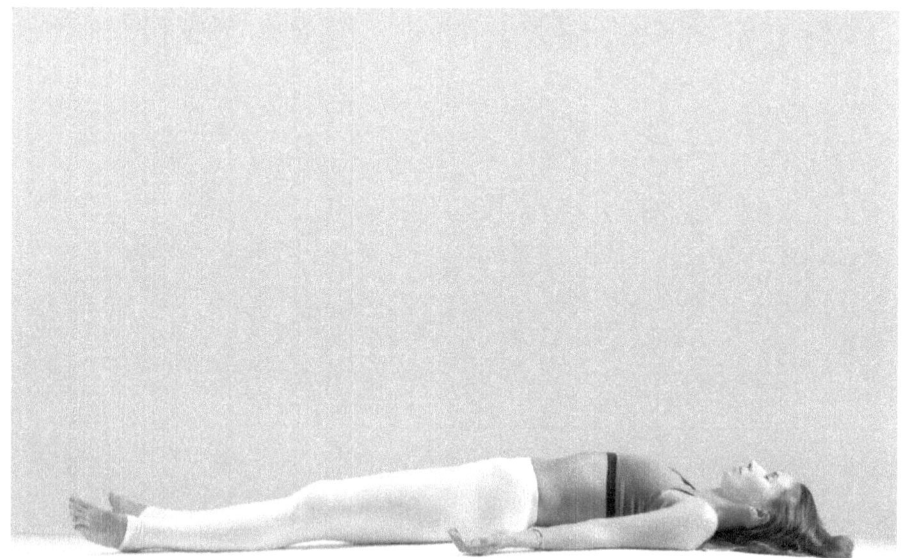

Corpse pose (Shavasana)

Many beginners thought that Shavasana pose is easy, but more experienced yoga students know that Shavasana can actually be the most challenging and beneficial of all the poses. That's because the essence of Shavasana is to relax the mind and body while remaining present and maintaining awareness.

Shavasana helps you relax, causing a lowered heart rate, a sense of calm, and a decreased release of stress hormones, like adrenaline and cortisol. It makes us feel good. And that was just what we wanted. Now we can approach everyday problems and challenges and solve them using our calm mind.

MEDITATION PRACTICE

In order to have a successful meditation practice, you need regular, daily exercise, choose to just sit quietly and watch what happens. For that time, ignore your phone, don't answer the doorbell, don't add another item to your to-do list in your mind. Just sit and observe your thoughts as they come and pass through your mind. You will find it very hard, if not impossible, to have even half a minute of having a calm mind. It is only possible if you are determined and committed.

It is best to simply add it to the end of your daily yoga exercises, your asana practice. You can choose to practice meditation in some other part of the day, but the important thing is that you find a time that works best for you. Be patient; do not rush your practice. Soon, you will be able to have longer and longer sessions, and you will feel real benefits. To start, even 5 to 10 minutes is enough. You will probably be surprised by how difficult it is to sit quietly for "only" 10 minutes. Later, try to lengthen your meditation practice by 5 minutes every week until you reach your desired length. It can be anything from 20 to 60 minutes a day—or more if you can spare the time.

Almost all people that practice yoga also practices some form of meditation. Often, it is just a part of their yoga practice, but also as a separate practice for achieving their peace of mind. So over time, practitioners of yoga tend to seek some more complex meditation practices and to go deeper into the philosophy behind the techniques of meditation.

When and Where to Practice

Try to meditate at the same time and in the same place every day. This place should be quiet, a place where you will not be disturbed. If this is not available to you, it is essential to have in mind that you can meditate in other circumstances. It is not a reason to quit.

Some people are the most relaxed and ready to meditate in the morning. It helps them start the day with a positive mind. Evening meditation is more suitable for others because it calms their mind before sleeping at night.

Meditation Postures

Sitting on the floor is the most common meditation posture. You can also do walking or standing meditation. The only essential things are maintaining proper position and staying focused for the entire time.

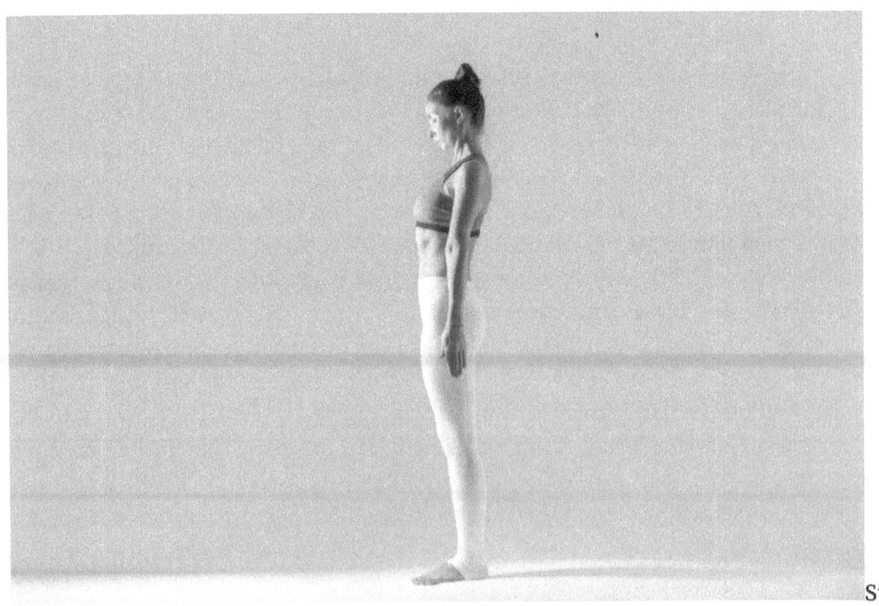

anding pose (Tadasana)

Standing

Standing is another meditation practice that you can use in combination with sitting meditation, to rest your body. It can be used as a complete practice in case you want to additionally build physical, mental, and spiritual strength. Stand with your feet about a hip's distance apart. Don't lock your knees, and let your arms rest comfortably at your sides. Your shoulders should be pulled back and down, chest open, neck long, head floating on top, and chin parallel to the floor. You can keep your eyes opened or closed.

Walking

It is one of the most widely used postures. You should walk slowly and consciously and focus on each step. Let your arms move freely at your sides. Your breath should be in synchronization with your footsteps.

Choose a quiet place. Focus on the individual parts of your steps: how you lift your foot, how you move it forward, how you put it back on the ground. Your pace should be moderate, and you should have enough space to make about 15 to 30 steps in one line. Then, you stop and turn. It is essential to make every move consciously, contemplating the movement in your mind. This involvement in your steps is your meditation practice. Often, practitioners combine walking and sitting meditation in successive sessions, sitting down for 30 minutes, then walking for 30 minutes, and so on.

Sitting

You can meditate while sitting on the floor or on a chair—whichever works for you. It is important to keep the spine upright, and the body relaxed. If you are sitting on the floor, in the beginning, you can assume for the basic Cross-Legged Pose (Sukhasana). If you are very flexible, you can sit down in Lotus Pose (Padmasana). You can also sit and kneel on a small, slanted wooden bench. Place your hands comfortably on your lap, knees, or thighs. Your palms can be up or down.

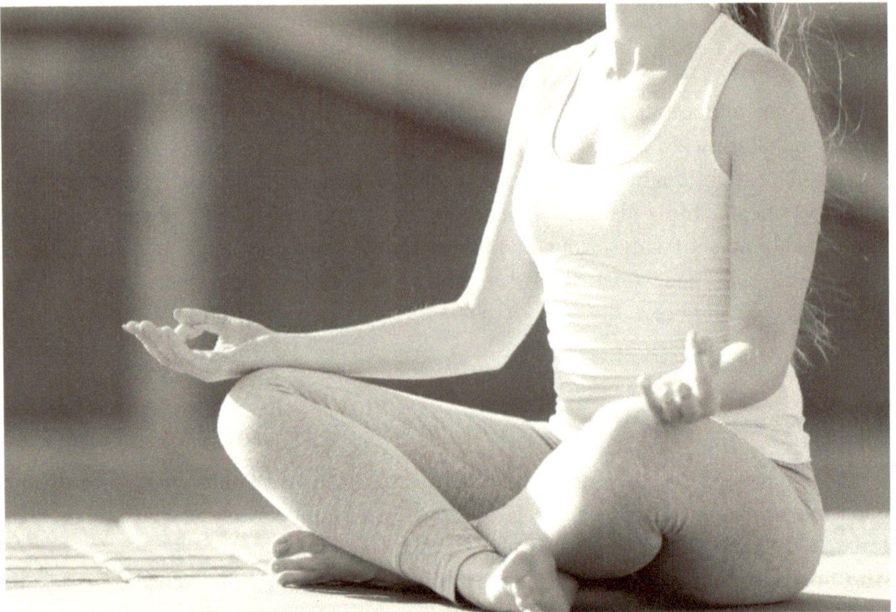

Cross-Legged Pose (Sukhasana)

Lying Down

It is also common to finish your yoga practice with lying-down meditation (Shavasana). In that case, be sure to assume a comfortable position and have the appropriate support under your head and knees if needed. Lie down on your back with your arms at your sides, palms facing upward. Your body needs to be fully relaxed. Your eyes can be open or closed, depending on if you feel you might fall asleep. It is a less physically challenging pose, but it requires more mental strength to remain awake and focused.

Methods of Meditation

The most common method of meditation is focusing on your breath. It is very convenient because it is always there for us. In the Buddhist tradition, this is the standard method of meditation. It is the simple observation of your breath as you inhale and exhale. In the beginning, you can count your inhalations and exhalations, and later, you will get accustomed to just observing various sensations that your breathing produces. In other teachings and traditions, there are additional methods and styles of meditation. In advanced stages, you will be able to observe your whole body and how it reacts to every breath you take.

Observing physical sensations is another way to meditate. You should do the same as you would when concentrating on your breaths. You can follow the sweat on your palms, the weight of your body pressing against the floor, the back pain from sitting for too long... You can also observe your emotions. Stick to your focus for the whole meditation practice. This method of meditation practice is more challenging than focusing on your breath, so it is not recommended for complete beginners. As a beginner, you can instead use mantras and visualizations together with concentrating on your breathing. In the end, you will need to find for yourself what helps develop the calmness of your mind the most.

Mantra, or silently or audibly repeating a word or phrase, is another ubiquitous method of meditation. You must choose a word or phrase that is calming to you, such as "peace," "love," or "joy."

You can use affirmations as well when you breathe out. If you repeat to yourself a phrase like "I feel relaxed, I feel peaceful," then you can calm your mind and meditate. Other options include using a recording of chants or listening to relaxing music.

You can also do visualizations, or you could imagine your favorite spot in nature with your eyes closed. You can direct your gaze toward an object in front of you. You can even possibly choose a lit candle, a flower, or a picture of a deity.

Once you find what works for you, you'll want to maintain that practice indefinitely, but in the beginning, try to give various methods a chance for some time, like one month, to be sure what is best for you.

Your thoughts will wander. It happens to most experienced meditators, so this should not discourage you. You will, in that case, just gently remind yourself to go back to your object of meditation and start over. It will happen again and again. This is also how you improve your focus and willpower.

BECOMING PEACEFUL WITH YOUR THOUGHTS

Find your own meditation style.

It is not easy to have an empty mind. This is true not only for beginners but also for everyone who has really tried to achieve this goal. In this book, we have some tools that can help you get started, like with guided meditation practice, books, or friends that are already practicing meditation. It is usual to start by focusing on your breath and then gain focus. In the later stages of your practice, you can experiment with other types of meditation and find out which ones work for you. Usually, people combine a few different types of meditation practice, depending on how they feel that day.

Get rid of distractions.

Be sure to find a quiet place, but if one is not available to you, do not worry. You can create your own quiet place in time, in your mind. Turn off your mobile phone, forget about things that happened yesterday, and, most importantly, do not think about what you must do today. Do not let distractions defeat you. It is not easy, but in time, it will get more and more manageable. Assume the posture of your choice and then allow your breath and energy to flow freely.

Establish a habit.

Try to meditate regularly at the same time and place every day. But this is not a must. Just remember to practice every day, making it a habit, almost like you brush your teeth or take a morning shower. You will find, in time, that your mind will ask for your daily meditation practice itself.

Be patient.

Success will not come overnight; it never does. Almost every experienced meditator will say to you that establishing a practice is merely showing up every day. This is not entirely true. You need to put some effort into your practice and have patience. It may take months before you can really feel some progress. If you are genuinely committed to meditation practice, then the results will eventually show themselves. Do not quit.

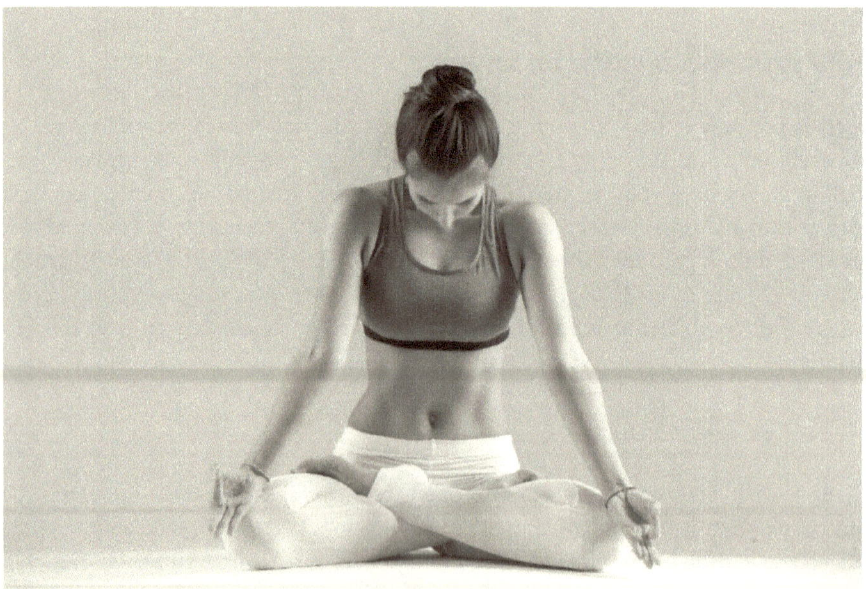

Lotus Pose (Padmasana)

Find the joy.

I think the most important thing is to find joy in meditation. We are all doing this because we want to feel better. We want to feel peace of mind, happiness, and joy. Without this, it really isn't worth it. Give it a chance to become your true nature and to sink deeply into your everyday life. Have an open mind. You will find how small, daily wins contribute so much to your whole mental health. You will see how small losses are not worth stressing out about. Let go of toxic people and look at dark situations with optimism. Your life will become much better. You will start to feel joy.

Just start meditating.

The first step can be the hardest. If you have trouble finding the right time, right place, or right mood to start, maybe it would be better to join a group or class. Later, you can broaden this practice with some guided video meditations, or you could just try to sit alone again. Make this first step into a mindfulness practice. Give it a fair chance.

Challenges You May Face

When you start your practice, and even before that, you may face some of your fears or worries. Some people are afraid to be alone with their own thoughts. It is possible that, during meditation, some thoughts that you were trying to avoid will emerge. But the purpose of mindfulness meditation is actually to train your mind to recognize them as bad habits and how to learn to let them go.

There is no point in dwelling in the past. You cannot change it.

You can learn from your past, of course. Just do not let the past become the source of your stress today. The same applies to the fear of an uncertain future. It may never come. Do plan and prepare for the future, but do not let it preoccupy your mind. This fear can be replaced by full mindfulness that anchors you in the present.

Your mind always wanders around. It cannot stand still, but this is not a reason to worry. Everybody's mind does just that. The way to calm your mind is to let go of preconceived notions and expectations. Don't expect to instantly feel better or to solve all your troubles. Just dedicate the next 5 to 20 minutes to meditation. During meditation, as good or bad feelings arise, let go of them. They are just distractors from the present moment. Your goal is to stay neutral and objective. When those thoughts occur, just gently steer your focus to the breath or the object of meditation in your practice. Do that as many times as needed. In time, you will need to do this less and less, and you will start to feel all the benefits of your meditation practice.

Is It Working for You?

You mustn't have any expectations for your meditation practice. The goal is to be in the moment and to let go of your regrets about the past or your expectations for the future. Also, we are not used to sitting on the floor for a long time. We might get uncomfortable or even feel some pain. You can change the position in that case, but try to make that choice consciously with intention and to not do it too often. Meditation shouldn't cause you to feel stressed or physically uncomfortable. Try to relax, but if you still feel uncomfortable, you can reduce the length of your meditation. You can even change your position from sitting to standing, for example.

There is also the consideration of a teacher. A good teacher can help, but you should not forget that no one can directly help someone else.

Personally, I find that I have better meditation practice when in a group. Try to join a community of yogis or meditators. There are many groups with different meditation techniques, even goals, so there is a wide range of choices for you. You may find that meditation retreats work for you. I find them enlightening. Do not quit easily, and be patient and consistent. You will probably find the results to be lifechanging.

YOU NEED TO PRACTICE EVERY DAY

There are many ways to achieve your peace of mind. Meditation is one of the most helpful tools for doing just that. It does not matter which technique or method you choose. It is important to be persistent in your practice and patient when expecting the results. You really must practice (almost) every day to be able to have some effects. It can be hard at the beginning, but once you develop the habit, it gets much more comfortable, and it becomes part of who you are.

The present moment is the only place and time where you can decide what your answer will be to what life puts before you. The past is irreversibly behind you; there is no more than that, except for the memories in your mind and this very moment. The future doesn't exist either, except as thoughts in the present moment. So, all that exists is only now created through a mixture of causes and conditions, most of which you cannot control. The one and only choice that is under your control is your reaction here and now.

When you notice that your mind begins to preoccupy you with thoughts of the future or the past, gently restore it to the present moment by looking closely at the sky or the people around you.

Even though the reward is valuable, it is a big challenge as well. Thus, it is necessary to arm yourself with patience.

CONCLUSION

Thank you again for reading this book! I hope this book was able to help you to learn how to improve your mental health through the practice of mindfulness meditation, to create your inner peace, and to make your life better.

You can find my other work on Amazon and other stores, as a paperback, but also as E-Books:

1) Mindfulness Meditation: A Beginner's Guide to Yoga Meditation

2) Procrastination Cure: How to Use Mindfulness Meditation to Stop Procrastinating

3) Procrastination: How To Stop Wasting Your Time And Be More Productive

4) Mindfulness: The Benefits of Meditation, a Beginner's Guide to Peace of Mind in Your Everyday Life

If you like this book, please follow me on:
Facebook https://www.facebook.com/gmposi/
Twitter https://twitter.com/george_posi
Instagram https://www.instagram.com/georgemposi
YouTube https://www.youtube.com/channel/UCmffykN4Iq8TY_1yyUWdoeA

Share how did you like my work on Facebook or Twitter with your friends!
Visit my blog site https://georgemposi.com

Finally, if you enjoyed this book, would you be kind enough to leave an honest review for it on Amazon.

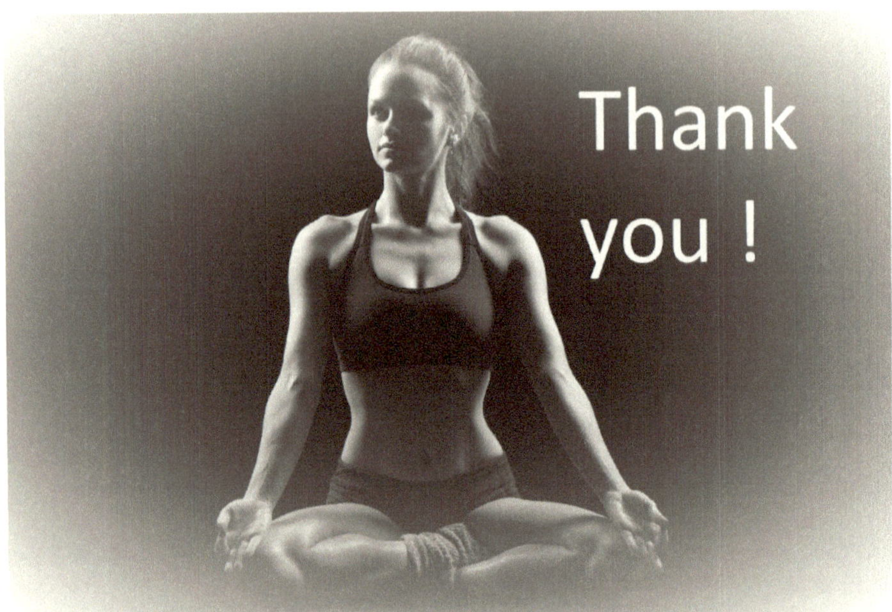

* Image Designed by Yanalya / Freepik

ABOUT THE AUTHOR

George M. Posi is an internet author and publisher and experienced entrepreneur. For the past 30 years, he has been the owner and manager of his own IT company. Five years ago, he started his journey towards mindfulness and began to seek new challenges. Then he promised himself that all business that he does must be done with respect and kindness to himself and to others.

George M. Posi started writing and publishing books as a way to reach as many people he can, to help others commit to this value in every area of their lives through self-development, including health, fitness, emotions, mindset, and spirituality.

He is grateful for all the experiences that he had in his life this first 55 years. All of those, positive and negative, helped him learn valuable life lessons. His life has since truly changed. His mission is to give back and serve others and to be a positive example of the unlimited possibilities that life offers for those that are genuinely committed to seeking mindfulness in their everyday activities.

Visit the website https://georgemposi.com, as well as YouTube channel Mindfulness Journey, where he openly and passionately shares all his experiences that have made a measurable difference to the quality of his life and will for yours as well.

Topics that George M. Posi writes about are Health and Fitness, Yoga, Mind and Beliefs, Emotions, Mission and Purpose, Productivity, Spirituality, and more...

www.ingramcontent.com/pod-product-compliance
Lightning Source LLC
Chambersburg PA
CBHW051135250726
48655CB00007B/3072